Military Medical Care: Questions and Answers

Don J. Jansen
Analyst in Defense Health Care Policy

January 2, 2014

Congressional Research Service

7-5700

www.crs.gov

RL33537

Summary

The primary objective of the military health system, which includes the Defense Department's hospitals, clinics, and medical personnel, is to maintain the health of military personnel so they can carry out their military missions and to be prepared to deliver health care during wartime. The military health system also covers dependents of active duty personnel, military retirees, and their dependents, including some members of the reserve components. The military health system provides health care services through either Department of Defense (DOD) medical facilities, known as "military treatment facilities" or "MTFs" as space is available, or through private health care providers. The military health system serves 9.7 million beneficiaries through care purchased from private providers as well as directly through a system of DOD military treatment facilities that currently includes some 56 hospitals and 365 clinics. It operates worldwide and employs some 58,369 civilians and 86,007 military personnel.

Since 1966, civilian care to millions of dependents and retirees (and retirees' dependents) has been provided through a program still known in law as the Civilian Health and Medical Program of the Uniformed Services (CHAMPUS), but more commonly known as TRICARE. TRICARE has four main benefit plans: a health maintenance organization option (TRICARE Prime), a preferred provider option (TRICARE Extra), a fee-for-service option (TRICARE Standard), and a Medicare wrap-around option (TRICARE for Life) for Medicare-eligible retirees. Other TRICARE plans include TRICARE Young Adult, TRICARE Reserve Select and TRICARE Retired Reserve. TRICARE also includes a pharmacy program and optional dental plans. Options available to beneficiaries vary by the beneficiary's duty status and location.

This report answers several frequently asked questions about military health care, including

- How is the military health system structured?
- What is TRICARE?
- What are the different TRICARE plans and who is eligible?
- What are the costs of military health care to beneficiaries?
- What is the relationship of TRICARE to Medicare?
- How does the Affordable Care Act affect TRICARE?
- What are the long-term trends in defense health care costs?
- What is the Medicare Eligible Retiree Health Care fund, which funds TRICARE for Life?

The Government Accountability Office (GAO) and the Congressional Budget Office (CBO) have also published important studies on the organization, coordination, and costs of the military health system, as well as its effectiveness addressing particular health challenges. The Office of the Assistant Secretary of Defense for Health Affairs Home Page, available at http://www.health.mil/, may also be of interest for additional information on the military health system. This report does not address issues specific to battlefield medicine, veterans, or the Veterans Health Administration. Veterans' health issues are addressed in CRS Report R42747, *Health Care for Veterans: Answers to Frequently Asked Questions*, by Sidath Viranga Panangala and Erin Bagalman.

Contents

Background 1

Questions and Answers 1
    1. How is the Military Health System Structured? 1
        Leadership 1
        Defense Health Agency 3
        TRICARE Regional Managed Health Care Support Contracts 3
    2. What is the Unified Medical Budget? 4
    3. What is the Medicare Eligible Retiree Health Care Fund (MERHCF)? 5
    4. What is TRICARE? 6
    5. Who Is Eligible to Receive Care? 7
    6. What are the Different TRICARE Plans? 7
        TRICARE Prime 7
        TRICARE Standard 8
        TRICARE Extra 8
        TRICARE Reserve Select 8
        TRICARE Retired Reserve 9
        TRICARE Young Adult 9
        TRICARE for Life 9
    7. How Much Does Military Health Care Cost Beneficiaries? 10
    8. What is the Pharmacy Benefits Program? 12
    9. What is the Extended Care Health Option (ECHO) Program? 14
    10. How Are Priorities for Care in Military Medical Facilities Assigned? 15
    11. What are the Long-Term Trends in Defense Health Costs? 16
    12. How Does the Patient Protection and Affordable Care Act Affect TRICARE? 19
    13. How Are Private Health Care Providers Paid? 19
    14. What Is the Relationship of DOD Health Care to Medicare? 20
        TRICARE and Medicare Payments to Providers and the Sustainable Growth Rate 20
        Medicare and TRICARE for Life 21
    15. What Medical Benefits are Available to Reservists? 21
    16. Have Military Personnel Been Promised Free Medical Care for Life? 22
    17. What is the Congressionally Directed Medical Research Program? 23
    18. Other Frequently Asked Questions 24
        Does TRICARE Cover Abortion? 24
        Does DOD Use Animals in Medical Research or Training? 25

Figures

Figure 1. FY2014 Unified Medical Budget Request ($billions) 5
Figure 2. Military Health System Eligible Beneficiaries (millions) 7
Figure 3. CBO Depiction of Funding for the MHS, by Category 17
Figure 4. CBO Depiction of Actual and Projected Costs for Military Health Care as a
    Share of DoD's Budget, 1990 to 2030 18

Tables

Table 1. Selected TRICARE Cost-Sharing Features 10
Table 2. Appropriation Levels by Fiscal Year (FY) for Selected CDMR Programs,
FY2007-FY2013 23

Contacts

Author Contact Information.. 25

Background

Since 1966, civilian healthcare to millions of service members' dependents and retirees (and retirees' dependents) has been provided through a program still known in law as the Civilian Health and Medical Program of the Uniformed Services (CHAMPUS), but more commonly known as TRICARE. The "TRI" in "TRICARE" originally referred to the three main main benefit plan options: a health maintenance organization option (TRICARE Prime), a preferred provider option (TRICARE Extra), and a fee-for-service option (TRICARE Standard). A Medicare wrap-around option (TRICARE for Life) for Medicare-eligible retirees was added in 2002. Other TRICARE plans include TRICARE Young Adult, TRICARE Reserve Select, and TRICARE Retired Reserve. TRICARE also includes a pharmacy program and optional dental plans. Options available to beneficiaries vary by the beneficiary's duty status and location.

The Government Accountability Office (GAO) and the Congressional Budget Office (CBO) have also published important studies on the organization, coordination, and costs of the military health system, as well as its effectiveness addressing particular health challenges. Another source of information is the Office of the Assistant Secretary of Defense for Health Affairs Home Page.[1]

Questions and Answers

1. How is the Military Health System Structured?

The Military Health System (MHS) restructured in the fall of 2013 and is now primarily administered by a new entity known as the Defense Health Agency (DHA). As described in the most recent DOD report to Congress on MHS administration, this resulted in the several new leadership organizations described below.[2] In addition, during 2013 a new round of regional managed care support contracts fully took effect.

Leadership

The Military Health System Executive Review (MHSER) serves as a senior-level forum for DOD leadership input into the strategic, transitional, and emerging issues. The MHSER advises the Office of the Secretary of Defense (SECDEF) and the Office of the Deputy Secretary of Defense (DEPSECDEF) about performance challenges and direction. The MHSER is chaired by the Under Secretary of Defense (Personnel and Readiness) (USD[P&R]), and includes the Principal Deputy Under Secretary of Defense (Personnel and Readiness), the Assistant Secretary of Defense (Health Affairs) (ASD[HA]), the service vice chiefs, military department assistant secretaries for manpower and reserve affairs, the Assistant Commandant of the Marine Corps, the Director of Program Analysis and Evaluation, the Principal Deputy Under Secretary of Defense (Comptroller), the Director of the Joint Staff, and the surgeons general (as ex-officio members).

---

[1] http://www health mil/

[2] Department of Defense, *Third Submission unders Section 731 of the National Defense Authorization Act for Fiscal year 2013: Plan for Reform of the Administration of the Military Health System*, October 25, 2013, pp. 1-6, http://www.tricare mil/tma/congressionalinformation/downloads/Military%20Health%20System%20Governance%20Reform%20Report.pdf.

The Senior Military Medical Action Council (SMMAC) is the highest governing body in the MHS. The SMMAC is chaired by the ASD(HA), and includes the Principal Deputy Assistant Secretary of Defense (Health Affairs) (PDASD[HA]), military department Surgeons General, DHA Director, Joint Staff Surgeon, and other attendees as required. The SMMAC presents enterprise-level guidance and operational issues for decision-making by the ASD(HA).

Reporting to the SMMAC is the Medical Deputies Action Group (MDAG), which ensures that actions are coordinated across the MHS and are in alignment with strategy, policies, directives, and initiatives of the MHS. The MDAG is chaired by the PDASD(HA), and includes the Deputy Surgeons General, DHA Deputy Director, and a Joint Staff Surgeon Representative.

Reporting to the MDAG are four supporting governing bodies:

- The Medical Operations Group (MOG) consists of the senior healthcare operations directors of the Service medical departments, the DHA Director of Healthcare Operations, and a Joint Staff Surgeon representative, with the chairmanship rotating among these members. The MOG carries out MDAG assigned tasks and provides a collaborative and transparent forum supporting enterprise-wide oversight of direct and purchased care systems focused on sustaining and improving the MHS.

- The Medical Business Operations Group (MBOG) consists of the senior resource managers of the Service medical departments and the DHA Director of Business Operations, with the chairmanship rotating among these members. The MBOG provides a forum for providing resource management input to the MDAG on direct and purchased care issues and initiatives focused on sustaining and improving the MHS.

- The Human Resources and Manpower Workgroup (HR&MANPOWER WG) consists of the senior human resources and manpower representatives from the Service medical departments and the DHA, with the chairmanship rotating among these members. The HR&MANPOWER WG supports centralized, coordinated policy execution, and guidance for development of coordinated human resources and manpower policies and procedures for the MHS.

- The Enhanced Multi-Service Markets (eMSM) Leadership Group. eMSMs are geographic MHS markets served by more than one military department under the direction of a designated Market Manager with enhanced authorities. The six eMSMs are:

1. Tidewater, Virginia
2. Puget Sound, Washington
3. Colorado Springs, Colorado
4. San Antonio, Texas
5. Oahu, Hawaii
6. National Capital Region

- The eMSM Leadership Group is composed of the six Market Managers, with the chairmanship rotating among these members. The eMSM Leadership Group provides a forum for eMSM Managers to discuss clinical and business issues, policies, performance standards, and opportunities.

Finally, the ASD(HA) is supported and advised by the Policy Advisory Council (PAC), composed of the Deputy Assistant Secretaries of Defense (Health Affairs), the DHA Deputy Director, the Deputy Surgeons General, and a representative of the Joint Staff. The PAC provides a forum for supporting MHS-wide policy development and oversight in a unified manner.

Defense Health Agency

On the operational side, the Defense Health Agency (DHA) is designated as a Combat Support Agency in order to ensure that the DHA remains focused on the primary mission of medical readiness, and is responsive to the Combatant Commanders through a formal oversight process established by the Chairman, Joint Chiefs of Staff. The Assistant Secretary of Defense for Health Affairs (ASD(HA)) will provide the Deputy Secretary of Defense with a detailed plan for implementing a shared services model within the military health system. A "shared services model" means that the DHA will assume responsibility for shared services, functions, and activities in the military health system, including the TRICARE program, pharmacy programs, medical education and training, medical research and development, health information technology, facility planning, public health, medical logistics, acquisition, budget, and resource management. The current Joint Task Force National Capital Region Medical (JTF CAPMED) will be assigned to an organization subordinate to the DHA that will be known as the National Capital Region.

The military health system serving 9.7 million beneficiaries through care purchased from private providers as well as directly through a system of DOD military treatment facilities that currently includes some 56 hospitals and 365 clinics. It operates worldwide and employs approximately 68,000 civilians and 86,000 military personnel. Direct care costs include the provision of medical care directly to beneficiaries, the administrative requirements of a large medical establishment, and maintaining a capability to provide medical care to combat forces in case of hostilities. Civilian providers under contract to DOD have constituted a major portion of the defense health reconstruction in recent years.

TRICARE Regional Managed Health Care Support Contracts

TRICARE is administered through managed care support contracts in three regions:

- TRICARE North Region covering Connecticut, Delaware, the District of Columbia, Illinois, Indiana, Kentucky, Maine, Maryland, Massachusetts, Michigan, New Hampshire, New Jersey, New York, North Carolina, Ohio, Pennsylvania, Rhode Island, Vermont, Virginia, West Virginia, Wisconsin, and portions of Iowa, Missouri, and Tennessee. The TRICARE North regional contractor is currently Health Net Federal Services.

- TRICARE South Region covering Alabama, Arkansas, Florida, Georgia, Louisiana, Mississippi, Oklahoma, South Carolina, and most of Tennessee and Texas. The TRICARE South regional contractor is currently Humana Military Health Services.

- TRICARE West Region covering Alaska, Arizona, California, Colorado, Hawaii, Idaho, most of Iowa, Kansas, Minnesota, most of Missouri, Montana, Nebraska,

Nevada, New Mexico, North Dakota, Oregon, South Dakota, portions of Texas, Utah, Washington, and Wyoming. The TRICARE West regional contractor is currently UnitedHealthcare.

These three contracts were re-competed in 2009, and after resolving bid protests, the new contracts known as "TRICARE Third Generation (T-3) Support Contracts" became operational between 2011 and 2012. Health care delivery under the new T-3 Contracts began April 1, 2011, for the North region with Health Net Federal Services. Humana Military Healthcare Services began health care delivery for TRICARE South region April 1, 2012. UnitedHealthcare began delivery of services to the TRICARE West region April 1, 2013.

2. What is the Unified Medical Budget?

ASD(HA) prepares and submits a unified medical budget, which includes resources for the medical activities under his or her control within the DOD. The unified medical budget includes funding for all fixed medical treatment facilities/activities, including such costs as real property maintenance, environmental compliance, minor construction, and base operations support. Funds for medical personnel and accrual payments to the Medicare Eligible Retiree Health Care Fund ((MERHCF)—see question "3. What is the Medicare Eligible Retiree Health Care Fund (MERHCF)?") are also included. The unified medical budget does not include resources associated with combat support medical units/activities. In these instances the funding responsibility is assigned to military service combatant or support commands.

Unified medical budget funding has traditionally been appropriated in several sources:

- The defense appropriations bill provides Operation and Maintenance (O&M), Procurement, and Research, Development, Test and Evaluation (RDT&E) funding under the heading "Defense Health Program."

- Funding for military medical personnel (doctors, corpsmen, and other health care providers) and TRICARE for Life accrual payments are generally provided in the defense appropriations bill under the "Military Personnel" (MILPERS) title.

- Funding for medical military construction (MILCON) is generally provided under the "Department of Defense" title of the military construction and veterans affairs bill.

- A standing authorization for transfers from the MERHCF to reimburse TRICARE for the cost of services provided to Medicare eligible retirees is provided by Section 1113 of title 10, United States Code (10 U.S.C. 1113).

- Costs of war-related military health care are generally funded through supplemental appropriations bills.

Other resources are made available to the military health system from third-party collections authorized by 10 U.S.C.1097b (b) and a number of other reimbursable program and transfer authorities. The President's budget typically refers to the unified medical budget request as its funding request for the military health system but only includes an exhibit for the DHP in the "Department of Defense—Military" chapter and exhibits for the MERHCF in the "Other Defense—Civil Programs" chapter of the Appendix volume. Medical MILCON and MILPERS request levels are generally found in DOD's budget submissions to Congress.

As illustrated in **Figure 1** below, the Obama Administration's FY2014 unified medical budget request[3] totals $49.4 billion and includes the following:

- $33.1 billion for the Defense Health Program (not including "Wounded, Ill, and Injured" funding);
- $8.5 billion for military personnel;
- $1.1 billion for medical military construction; and
- $6.7 billion for accrual payments to the MERHCF.

Much more detailed breakouts are available in budget exhibits published by the Department of Defense at http://www.budget.mil.

Figure 1. FY2014 Unified Medical Budget Request ($billions)

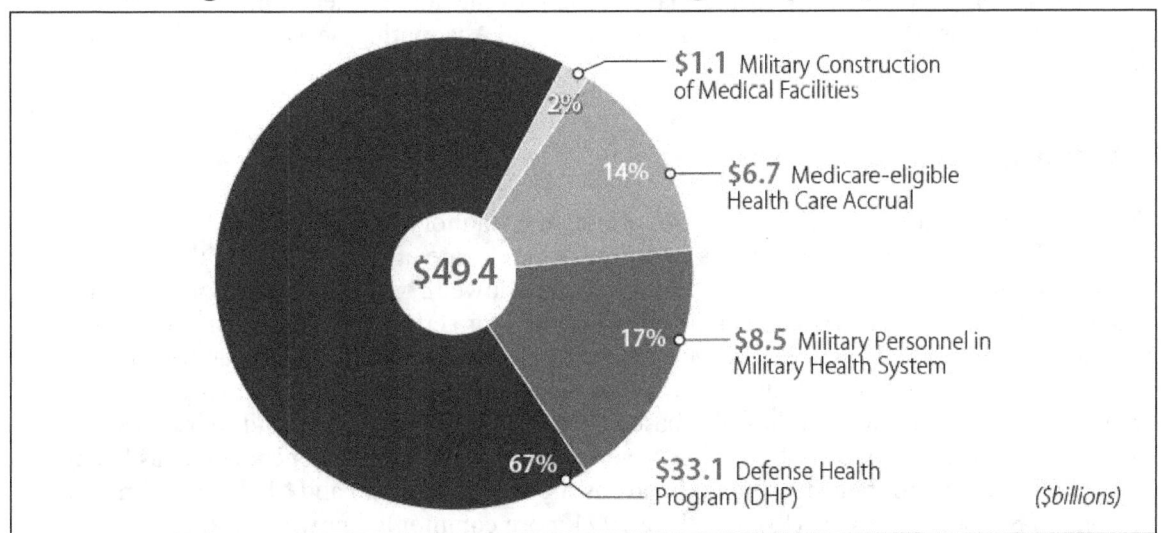

Source: Department of Defense FY2014 Budget Request Overview. Adapted by CRS Graphics.

3. What is the Medicare Eligible Retiree Health Care Fund (MERHCF)?

The Floyd D. Spence National Defense Authorization Act for FY2001(FY2001 NDAA),[4] directed the establishment of the Medicare-Eligible Retiree Health Care Fund to pay for Medicare-eligible retiree health care beginning on October 1, 2002, via a new program called TRICARE for Life. Prior to this date, care for Medicare-eligible beneficiaries was space-available care in Military Treatment Facilities (MTF). The MERHCF covers Medicare-eligible beneficiaries, regardless of age.

---

[3] Department of Defense, *FY 2014 Budget Request Overview*, April 2013, pp. 5-3, Figure 5-1, http://comptroller.defense.gov/defbudget/fy2014/FY2014_Budget_Request_Overview_Book.pdf
[4] P.L. 106-398

The FY2001 NDAA also established an independent three-member DOD Medicare-Eligible Retiree Health Care Board of Actuaries appointed by the Secretary of Defense. Accrual deposits into the Fund are made by the agencies who employ future beneficiaries (DOD and the other uniformed services including the Public Health Service, the Coast Guard, and the National Oceanic & Atmospheric Administration) based upon estimates of future TRICARE for Life expenses. Transfers out are made to the Defense Health Program based on estimates of the cost of care actually provided each year. As of September 30, 2011, the Fund had assets of over $163.6 billion to cover future expenses.[5]

The Board is required to review the actuarial status of the fund, to report annually to the Secretary of Defense, and to report to the President and Congress on the status of the fund at least every four years. The DOD Office of the Actuary provides all technical and administrative support to the Board. Within DOD, the Office of the Under Secretary of Defense for Personnel and Readiness, through the Office of the Assistant Secretary of Defense (OASD) for Health Affairs (HA), has as one of its missions operational oversight of the defense health program including management of the MERHCF. The Defense Finance and Accounting Service provides accounting and investment services for the Fund.

4. What is TRICARE?

The Dependents Medical Care Act of 1956[6] provided a statutory basis for dependents of active duty members, retirees, and dependents of retirees to seek care at MTFs. Prior to this time, authority for such care was fragmented. The 1956 act allowed DOD to contract for a health insurance plan for coverage of civilian hospital services for active duty dependents. Due to growing use of MTFs by eligible civilians and resource constraints, Congress adopted the Military Medical Benefits Amendments in 1966,[7] which allowed DOD to contract with civilian health providers to provide non-hospital-based care to eligible dependents and retirees. Since 1966, civilian care to millions of dependents and retirees (and retirees' dependents) has been provided through a program still known in law as the Civilian Health and Medical Program of the Uniformed Services (CHAMPUS), but since 1994 more commonly known as TRICARE.

TRICARE has four main benefit plans: a health maintenance organization option (TRICARE Prime), a preferred provider option (TRICARE Extra), a fee-for-service option (TRICARE Standard), and a Medicare wrap-around option (TRICARE for Life) for Medicare-eligible retirees. Other TRICARE plans include TRICARE Young Adult, TRICARE Reserve Select, and TRICARE Retired Reserve. These plans are described below. TRICARE also includes a Pharmacy program and optional dental plans. Options available to beneficiaries vary by the beneficiary's relationship to a sponsor, sponsor's duty status, and location.

---

[5] Department of Defense, *Fiscal Year 2011 Medicare-Eligible Retiree Health Care Fun Audited Financial Statements*, November 7, 2011, p. 5, http://comptroller.defense.gov/cfs/fy2011/12_Medicare_Eligible_Retiree_Health_Care_Fund/Fiscal_Year_2011_Medicare_Eligible_Retiree_Health_Care_Fund_Financial_Statements_and_Notes.pdf.

[6] P.L. 84-569.

[7] P.L 89-614.

5. Who Is Eligible to Receive Care?

Eligibility for TRICARE is determined by the uniformed services and reported to the Defense Enrollment Eligibility Reporting System (DEERS). All eligible beneficiaries must have their eligibility status recorded in DEERS.

TRICARE beneficiaries can be divided into two main categories: sponsors and dependents. Sponsors are usually active duty servicemembers, National Guard/Reserve members, or retired servicemembers. "Sponsor" refers to the person who is serving or who has served on active duty or in the National Guard or Reserves. "Dependent" is defined in 10 U.S.C. 1072 and includes a variety of relationships, for example, spouses (including same-sex spouses), children, and certain unremarried former spouses.

Figure 2 illustrates the major categories of eligible beneficiaries.

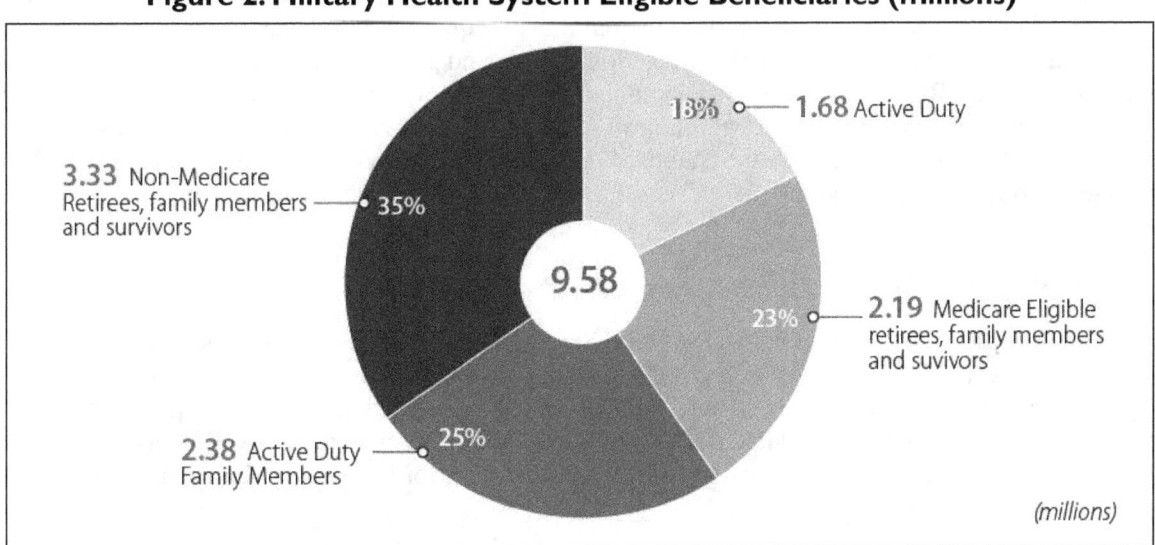

Figure 2. Military Health System Eligible Beneficiaries (millions)

Source: The President's Budget for FY2013, Appendix, "Department of Defense–Military Programs," p. 271. Adapted by CRS.

6. What are the Different TRICARE Plans?

TRICARE Prime

TRICARE Prime is a managed healthcare option similar to a health maintenance organization. Like such civilian arrangements, the plan's features include a primary healthcare provider (either a military or a civilian health care provider) who manages care and provides or facilitates referrals to specialists. Referrals generally are required for such visits. To participate, beneficiaries must enroll and pay an annual enrollment fee, which is similar to an annual premium. Eligible beneficiaries may choose to enroll at any time. Enrollees receive first priority for appointments at military health care facilities and pay less out of pocket than do beneficiaries who use the other TRICARE plans. TRICARE Prime does not have an annual deductible.

Active duty servicemembers are required to use TRICARE Prime. Both they and their family members, as well as surviving spouses (during the first three years) and surviving dependent children, are exempt from the annual enrollment fee. Retired servicemembers, their families, surviving spouses (after the first three years), eligible former spouses, and others are required to pay an annual enrollment fee, which is applied to the annual catastrophic out-of-pocket-limit. TRICARE Prime annual enrollment fees for military retirees were increased in FY2012 for new enrollees for the first time since the program began. Moving forward, under 10 U.S.C. 1097(e) TRICARE Prime enrollment fees will be subject to increases each fiscal year based on the annual retirement pay cost-of-living adjustment for the calendar year. For FY2013 (October 1, 2012– September 30, 2013) this enrollment fee is $269.28 for an individual and $538.56 for individual plus family coverage.

TRICARE Standard

TRICARE Standard is a traditional fee-for-service (FFS) option that does not require beneficiaries to enroll in order to participate. TRICARE Standard plan allows participants to use authorized out-of-network civilian providers, but it also requires users to pay higher out-of-pocket costs, generally 25% of the allowable charge for retirees and 20% for active duty family members. TRICARE Standard requires an annual deductible of $150/individual or $300/family for family members of sponsors at pay grades E-5 and above and $50/$100 for pay grades E-4 and below. Beneficiaries who use the Standard option must pay any difference between a provider's billed charges and the rate of reimbursement allowed under the plan.

TRICARE Extra

TRICARE Extra is also available to TRICARE Standard beneficiaries. It also has no formal enrollment requirement and mirrors a civilian preferred provider network. Network providers agree to accept a reduced payment from TRICARE and to file all claims for participants. By using network providers under TRICARE Extra, beneficiaries reduce their copayments, in general, to 20% of the allowable charge for retirees and 15% for active duty family members.

TRICARE Reserve Select

The TRICARE Reserve Select program was authorized by Section 701 of the Ronald W. Reagan National Defense Authorization Act for FY2005 (P.L. 108-375), which enacted 10 U.S.C. 1076d. TRICARE Reserve Select is a premium-based health plan available worldwide for qualified Selected Reserve members of the Ready Reserve and their families. Servicemembers are not eligible for TRICARE Reserve Select if they are on active duty orders, covered under the Transitional Assistance Management Program, or eligible for or enrolled in the Federal Employees Health Benefits Program (FEHBP) or currently covered under the FEHBP through a family member. TRICARE Reserve Select provides benefits similar to TRICARE Standard. The government subsidizes the cost of the program with members paying 28% of the cost of the program in the form of premiums. For calendar year 2013, premiums were $51.62 per month for member only coverage, and $195.81 per month for member and family coverage. For calendar year 2014, TRICARE Reserve Select premiums are $51.68 per month for member only coverage, and $204.29 per month for member and family coverage.

TRICARE Retired Reserve

Section 705 of the National Defense Authorization Act for FY2010 (P.L. 111-84) added a new 10 U.S.C. 1076e to authorize a TRICARE coverage option for so-called "gray area" reservists, those who have retired but are too young to draw retirement pay. The program established under this authority is known as TRICARE Retired Reserve. Previously, such individuals were not eligible for any TRICARE coverage. This is a premium-based health plan that qualified retired members of the National Guard and Reserve under the age of 60 may purchase for themselves and eligible family members. It is similar to TRICARE Reserve Select, but differs in that there is no government subsidy as there is with TRICARE Reserve Select. As such, retired Reserve Component members who elect to purchase TRICARE Retired Reserve must pay the full cost of the calculated premium plus an additional administrative fee. Retired Reserve Component personnel who elect to participate in TRICARE Retired Reserve become eligible for the same TRICARE Standard, TRICARE Extra, or TRICARE Prime options as active component retirees when the servicemember reaches age 60. Calendar year 2013 premiums for member only coverage were $402.11 per month and $969.10 per month for member-and-family plans. For calendar year 2014, TRICARE Retired Reserve premiums are $390.99 per month for member only coverage, and $956.65 per month for member and family coverage.

TRICARE Young Adult

Section 702 of the Ike Skelton National Defense Authorization Act for Fiscal Year 2011 (P.L. 111-383) added a new 10 U.S.C. 1110b, allowing unmarried children up to age 26, who are not otherwise eligible to enroll in an employer-sponsored plan, to purchase TRICARE coverage. The option established under this authority is known as "The TRICARE Young Adult Program." Unlike insurance coverage mandated by the Patient Protection and Affordable Care Act (P.L. 111-148), the TRICARE Young Adult Program provides individual coverage, rather than coverage under a family plan. A separate premium is charged. The law requires payment of a premium equal to the cost of the coverage as determined by the Secretary of Defense on an appropriate actuarial basis. For calendar year 2013 the monthly premium for a TRICARE Young Adult (TYA) Prime enrollment was $176 and $152 for a TYA Standard enrollment. For calendar year 2013 the monthly premium for a TRICARE Young Adult (TYA) Prime enrollment is $180 and $156 for a TYA Standard enrollment.

TRICARE for Life

TRICARE for Life was created as supplemental coverage to Medicare-eligible military retirees by Section 712 of the Floyd D. Spence National Defense Authorization Act for FY2001 (P.L. 106-398). TRICARE for Life functions as a secondary payer to Medicare, paying out-of-pocket costs for medical services covered under Medicare for beneficiaries who are entitled to Medicare Part A based on age, disability, or end-stage renal disease (ESRD). The beneficiaries are also eligible for medical benefits covered by TRICARE but not by Medicare. Prior to creation of the TRICARE for Life program, coverage for Medicare-eligible individuals was limited to space available care in military treatment facilities. In recognition of the requirement to enroll in Medicare Part B, TRICARE for Life cost-sharing for beneficiaries is limited and there is no enrollment charge.

In order to participate in TRICARE for Life, these TRICARE-eligible beneficiaries must enroll in and pay monthly premiums for Medicare Part B. TRICARE-eligible beneficiaries who are entitled to Medicare Part A based on age, disability, or ESRD, but decline Part B, lose eligibility for TRICARE benefits.[8] In addition, individuals who choose not to enroll in Medicare Part B upon becoming eligible may elect to do so later during an annual enrollment period; however, the Medicare Part B late enrollment penalty may apply.[9]

7. How Much Does Military Health Care Cost Beneficiaries?

Each TRICARE plan has its own cost-sharing arrangements based upon the sponsor's military status and where the care is received (military treatment facility, network provider, or non-network provider).

Active duty service members receive medical care at no cost. Active duty family members pay nothing out-of-pocket for any type of care unless using the point-of-service option. The point-of-service option (which allows eligible Prime beneficiaries to pay a fee to access authorized providers for routine or urgent care without a referral) has an annual $300 outpatient care deductible for individual coverage and $600 for family coverage. After the deductible is met, beneficiaries who use the point of service option pay 50% of the TRICARE-allowable charge as a cost-share.

The tables below illustrate selected beneficiary cost-share arrangements.

Table 1. Selected TRICARE Cost-Sharing Features

	TRICARE Prime	TRICARE Extra/Standard
Annual Enrollment Fee	Enrollment is required. There is no enrollment fee for active duty families. Retirees, their families and all others must pay annual enrollment fees to participate. For enrollments in fiscal year 2014, the fee is: Individual: $273.84 per year Family: $547.68 per year	None. Enrollment is not required.

---

[8] 10 U.S.C. §1086(d).

[9] CRS Report R40082, *Medicare: Part B Premiums*, by Patricia A. Davis

	TRICARE Prime	**TRICARE Extra/Standard**
Annual Deductible	No annual deductible unless you are using the point-of-service option: $300/Individual $600/Family Note: Active duty service members can't use the point-of-service option.	Active duty family members (sponsor rank E-4 and below): $50/Individual $100/Family Active duty family members (sponsor rank E-5 and above): $150/Individual $300/Family All others: $150/Individual $300/Family Note: The annual deductible is waived for Guard/Reserve family members whose sponsor was activated in support of a contingency operation.
Outpatient Visit	Network Provider: Active duty service members: $0 Active duty family members: $0 All others: $12 per visit Non-network Provider: With Primary Care Manager (PCM) referral: Same as network provider costs Without PCM referral: Point-of-service fees apply Note: Active duty service members may not use the point-of-service option.	Network Provider (Extra option): Active duty family members: 15% of negotiated fee after the annual deductible is met All others: 20% of negotiated fee after the annual deductible is met Non-network Provider (Standard option): Active duty family members: 20% of allowable charges after the annual deductible is met All others: 25% allowable charges after the annual deductible is met
Maximum Annual Out-of-Pocket Charge (Catastrophic Cap)	Active duty families: $1,000 per family, per fiscal year National Guard and Reserve families: $1,000 per family, per fiscal year Retired families (and all others): $3,000 per family, per fiscal year	Same as under Prime.

Source: TRICARE web site: http://www.tricare.mil/Welcome/ComparePlans.aspx

Notes: Current as of October 1, 2013.

8. What is the Pharmacy Benefits Program?

The Pharmacy Benefits Program is an adjunct to the various TRICARE plan options. Under this program, TRICARE beneficiaries are able to obtain prescription drugs through military treatment facilities, retail drug stores, and a national mail order plan. The Pharmacy Benefit Program is authorized under 10 U.S.C. 1074g.

The Pharmacy Benefits Program is required to maintain a formulary of pharmaceutical agents (hereinafter also referred to as "drugs" or "medications") in the complete range of therapeutic classes. This is known as the "Uniform Formulary." Selection of drugs for inclusion on the formulary is based on the relative clinical and cost effectiveness of the agents in each class.[10] The law further specifies that the formulary is to be maintained and updated by a Pharmacy and Therapeutics Committee whose members are composed of representatives of both military treatment facility pharmacies and health care providers.[11] The Pharmacy and Therapeutics Committee meets at least quarterly and its minutes are publicly available.[12] A Uniform Formulary Beneficiary Advisory (UFBA) is required to review and comment on formulary recommendations presented by the Pharmacy and Therapeutics Committee prior to those recommendations going to the Executive Director of TRICARE for approval. The UFBBA is composed of representatives of nongovernmental organizations and associations that represent the views and interests of a large number of eligible covered beneficiaries, contractors responsible for the TRICARE retail pharmacy program, contractors responsible for the national mail-order pharmacy program, and TRICARE network providers.[13]

Prescriptions Filled through Military Treatment Facilities

At a military treatment facility pharmacy, TRICARE beneficiaries may fill prescriptions from any provider, civilian or military, without a copayment. Military treatment facilities are required to stock a subset of the Uniform Formulary known as the "Basic Core Formulary." Additional pharmaceutical agents on the Uniform Formulary may also be carried by individual military treatment facilities in order to meet local requirements. Non-formulary drugs are generally not available through military treatment facilities. Certain Uniform Formulary covered pharmaceuticals, however, may not be carried due to national contracts with pharmaceutical manufactures.[14] DOD's Pharmacoeconomics Center collaborates with the Defense Supply Center Philadelphia (DSCP) in coordination with the Department of Veterans Affairs (VA) Pharmacy Benefits Management Strategic Health Group and the VA National Acquisition Center in Hines, Illinois, in developing contracting strategies and technical evaluation factors for national pharmaceutical contracting initiatives.

Prescriptions Filled through Retail Pharmacies

---

[10] 10 U.S.C. 1074g(a)(2)(A).

[11] 10 U.S.C. 1074g(b).

[12] Available at the Department of Defense Pharmacoeconomic Center web site: http://www.pec ha.osd.mil/.

[13] ibid.

[14] Office of the Assistant Secretary of Defense (Health Affairs), Memorandum subject "TRICARE Pharmacy Benefit Program Formulary Management" dated December 22, 2004. Accessed February 27, 2013, at http://pec ha.osd mil/P&T/PDF/04-032.pdf.

TRICARE beneficiaries also may fill prescriptions through retail pharmacy drug stores. DOD contracts for a TRICARE pharmacy benefit manager to administer both the retail and mail order options. The services provided by this contractor are known as "TPharm." The current contract, awarded in 2008, is with Express Scripts, Inc. (Express Scripts). Among other things, Express Scripts maintains a national network of retail pharmacies for DOD that beneficiaries may use without having to file a claim for reimbursement. Beneficiaries may also use non-network pharmacies. However, at non-network pharmacies, beneficiaries pay the full price of the medication up front and then file a claim for reimbursement.

DOD requires prescriptions to be filled, when available, with generic drugs. These are defined as those medications approved by the Food and Drug Administration that are clinically the same as brand-name medications. Brand-name drugs that have a generic equivalent are only dispensed after the prescribing provider completes a clinical assessment that indicates the brand-name drug should be used in place of the generic medication and approval is granted by Express Scripts.

Currently, the copayments for non-active duty beneficiaries for a 30-day supply of medicine filled through a network pharmacy are $5 for generic formulary medications, $17 for brand-name formulary medications, and $44 for non-formulary medications, unless medical necessity is established. Copayments for prescriptions filled at non-network pharmacies vary based on the TRICARE plan covering the beneficiary and the type of prescription:

- Active duty service members receive full reimbursement after they file a claim.

- All others enrolled in a TRICARE Prime option pay a 50% cost share after a deductible is met. This deductible is $50 per person and $100 per family per year for service members in pay grades E1–E4 and $150 per person and $300 per family for all other beneficiaries.

- After annual deductibles of $150 per person and $300 per family are met, beneficiaries using Standard/Extra, TRICARE Reserve Select, TRICARE Retired Reserve or TRICARE Young Adult for a 30-day supply pay $17 or 20% of the total cost, whichever is greater, for formulary generic or brand name drugs, and, $44 or 20% of the total cost, whichever is greater, for non-formulary medications.[15]

- Under recent legislation,[16] pharmaceuticals paid for by DOD that are provided by network retail pharmacies to TRICARE beneficiaries are subject to federal pricing standards. These pricing standards were established under the Veterans Health Care Act of 1992.[17] This act established federal ceiling prices for covered pharmaceuticals, which require a minimum 24% discount off non-federal average manufacturing prices. As a result, the overall growth of retail prescription drug costs for DOD has slowed.[18]

---

[15] TRICARE web site accessed February 26, 2013, http://www.tricare mil/pharmacycosts.

[16] Section 703 of the National Defense Authorization Act for Fiscal Year 2008 (P.L. 110-181).

[17] P.L. 102-585, codified at 38 U.S.C. 8126.

[18] Department of Defense, "Evaluation of the TRICARE Program, Fiscal Year 2012 Report to Congress," March 19, 2012, p. 75. Accessed February 26, 2013, at
http://www.tricare mil/tma/congressionalinformation/downloads/TRICARE%20Evaluation%20Report%20-%20FY12.pdf.

Prescriptions Filled by Mail Order

TRICARE beneficiaries may arrange for home delivery of prescription drugs through the mail by registering with Express Scripts. The copayments for a 90-day supply of medication filled by mail order are currently $13 for brand-name formulary medications, and $43 for non-formulary medications, unless medical necessity is established. Copayments for home delivery of generic drugs were eliminated effective October 1, 2011, as an incentive for beneficiaries to use the home delivery service. DOD negotiates prices with pharmaceutical manufacturers for the drugs dispensed by mail order that are considerably lower than those for drugs dispensed through retail pharmacies. In November 2009, DOD launched a campaign to educate beneficiaries on the benefits of home delivery services. Use of home delivery by TRICARE beneficiaries increased by 17% from FY2009 to FY2011.[19]

Copayment Adjustments

The Secretary of Defense is authorized to set and adjust copayment requirements for the pharmacy program under 10 U.S.C. 1074g; however, Section 712 of the National Defense Authorization Act for FY2013 amended this provision to limit any copayment increases in FY2014 to FY2022 to the percentage by which retirement pay is increased that year.

9. What is the Extended Care Health Option (ECHO) Program?

The Extended Care Health Option (ECHO) is a program for qualified beneficiaries that supplements TRICARE. It provides benefits that are not covered by TRICARE, such as assistive services, equipment, in-home respite care services and special education for qualifying mental or physical conditions. Qualifying conditions include:

- Diagnosis in an infant or toddler of a neuromuscular developmental condition or other condition expected to precede a diagnosis of moderate or severe mental retardation or serious physical disability;
- Extraordinary physical or psychological conditions causing the beneficiary to be homebound;
- Moderate or severe mental retardation;
- Multiple disabilities, and;
- Severe physical disability.

Access to ECHO benefits requires registration. To use ECHO, qualified beneficiaries must be enrolled in the Exceptional Family Member Program (EFMP) as provided by the sponsor's branch of service and be registered through the ECHO case manager in the applicable TRICARE region. There are no enrollment fees, but there is a monthly cost share based on the sponsor's pay grade. For 2013, monthly costs range from $25 for pay grades E-1 through E-4 to $250 for pay

---

[19] Department of Defense, "Evaluation of the TRICARE Program, Fiscal Year 2012 Report to Congress," March 19, 2012, p. 74. Accessed February 26, 2013, at
http://www.tricare.mil/tma/congressionalinformation/downloads/TRICARE%20Evaluation%20Report%20-%20FY12.pdf.

grade O-10. The total TRICARE cost share for all ECHO benefits combined, excluding the ECHO Home Health Care (EHHC) benefit, is $36,000 per covered beneficiary per fiscal year.[20]

EHHC provides medically-necessary skilled services to those ECHO beneficiaries who are homebound and generally require more than 28 to 35 hours per week of home health services or respite care. The EHHC benefit is only available in the United States, District of Columbia, Puerto Rico, the U.S. Virgin Islands, and Guam. Coverage for the EHHC benefit is capped on an annual basis. The cap is limited to the maximum fiscal year amount TRICARE would pay if the beneficiary resided in a skilled nursing facility. This amount is based on the beneficiary's geographic location.

ECHO qualified beneficiaries include:

- Active duty family members;
- Family members of activated National Guard/Reserve members;
- Family members who are covered under the Transitional Assistance Management Program;
- Children or spouses of former service members who are victims of abuse and qualify for the Transitional Compensation Program; and
- Family members of deceased active duty sponsors while they are considered "transitional survivors."

ECHO is authorized under 10 U.S.C. 1079.

10. How Are Priorities for Care in Military Medical Facilities Assigned?

Active duty personnel, military retirees, and their respective dependents are not afforded equal access to care in military medical facilities. Active duty personnel receive top priority access and are "entitled" to health care in a military medical facility (10 U.S.C. 1074).

According to 10 U.S.C. 1076, dependents of active duty personnel are "entitled, upon request, to medical and dental care" on a space-available basis at a military medical facility. 10 U.S.C. 1074 states that "a member or former member of the uniformed services who *is* entitled to retired or retainer pay ... may, upon request, be given medical and dental care in any facility of the uniformed service" on a space-available basis.

This language entitles active duty dependents to medical and dental care subject to space-available limitations. No such entitlement or "right" is provided to retirees or their dependents. Instead, retirees and their dependents may be given medical and dental care, subject to the same space-available limitations. This language gives active duty personnel and their dependents priority in receiving medical and dental care at any facility of the uniformed services over military members entitled to receive retired pay and their dependents. The policy of providing active duty dependents priority over retirees in the receipt of medical and dental care in any

---

[20] For additional information please see the ECHO web page at http://www.tricare.mil/echo.

facility of the uniformed services has existed in law since at least September 2, 1958 (P.L. 85-861).

Since the establishment of TRICARE and pursuant to the Defense Authorization Act of FY1996 (P.L. 104-106), DOD has established the following basic priorities (with certain special provisions):

> Priority 1: Active-duty servicemembers;
>
> Priority 2: Active-duty family members who are enrolled in TRICARE Prime;
>
> Priority 3: Retirees, their family members and survivors who are enrolled in TRICARE Prime;
>
> Priority 4: Active-duty family members who are not enrolled in TRICARE Prime;
>
> Priority 5: All other eligible persons.

The priority is given to active duty dependents to help them obtain care easily, and thus make it possible for active duty members to perform their military service without worrying about health care for their dependents. This is particularly important for active duty personnel who may be assigned overseas or aboard ship and separated from their dependents. As retirees are not subject to such imposed separations, they are considered to be in a better position to see that their dependents receive care, if care cannot be provided in a military facility. Thus, the role of health care delivery recognizes the unique needs of the military mission. The role of health care in the military is qualitatively different, and, therefore, not necessarily comparable to the civilian sector.

The benefits available to servicemembers or retirees, which require comparatively little or no contributions from the beneficiaries themselves, are considered by some to be a more generous benefit package than is available to civil servants or to most people in the private sector. Retirees may also be eligible to receive medical care at Department of Veterans Affairs (VA) medical facilities.

11. What are the Long-Term Trends in Defense Health Costs?

Even as the number of active duty personnel in DOD declines over the next few years, costs associated with the military health system are expected to grow. Total military health system costs (excluding TRICARE for Life) increased between FY2009 and FY2011 for inpatient and outpatient services but declined for prescription drugs, due to the FY2008 NDAA requirement that the TRICARE retail pharmacy program be subject to the same pricing standards as other federal agencies.

DOD's FY2013 appropriations request for the Defense Health Program and the Medical Eligible Retiree Health Fund was approximately 7.4% of DOD's total FY2013 appropriations request.[21] The Congressional Budget Office (CBO) projects that the cost of the military health care system will grow from $51 billion in FY2013 (higher than DOD's FY2013 budget request of $47 billion)

---

[21] Comptroller, Department of Defense. National Defense Budget Estimates for FY2013, March 2012. Table 3-1, Reconciliation of Authorization, Appropriation, TOA and BA, by Program, by Appropriation. pp. 36-44, http://comptroller.defense.gov/defbudget/fy2013/FY13_Green_Book.pdf.

to $65 billion by FY2017 and $95 billion by FY2030.[22] Over the Future Years Defense Plan
(FYDP) period from FY2013 to FY2017, CBO's projection has average annual growth of 6.0%,
compared with 2.6% in DOD's projection. Over the entire FY2013-FY2030 period, CBO
estimates the real (inflation-adjusted) growth rates in cost per user in the military health system
would average 5.5% per year for pharmaceuticals, 4.7% for purchased care and contracts, and
3.3% for direct care and administration. Please see **Figure 3** and **Figure 4** below. Overall, DOD
forecasts expect Defense Health Program costs to increase by 3.4% in FY2014, 3.35% in
FY2015, 3.6% in FY2016, and 3.9% in FY2017, in constant FY2013 dollars.[23]

Figure 3. CBO Depiction of Funding for the MHS, by Category

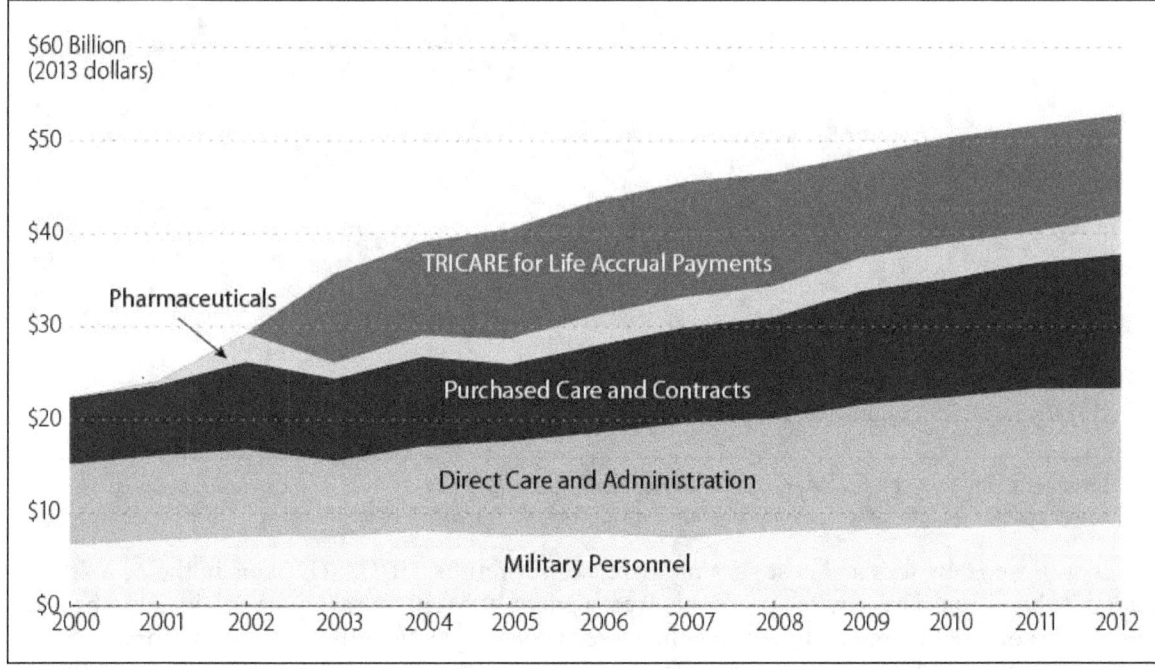

Source: Carla Tighe Murray, *Approaches to Reduce Federal Spending on the Defense Health System*, Congressional Budget Office, July 31, 2013, p. 3, http://www.cbo.gov/publication/44393.

This cost growth stems in part from general inflation in the cost of health care, as well as an
increasing percentage of care being provided to retirees and their dependents. DOD estimates that
care provided to retirees and their dependents will make up over 65% of DOD health care costs
by 2015, up from 43% in 1999. A recent CBO analysis concludes that this increasing proportion
of retirees participating in TRICARE is driven by "low out-of-pocket expenses for TRICARE
beneficiaries (many of whose copayments, deductibles, and maximum annual out-of-pocket
payments have remained unchanged or have decreased since the mid-1990s), combined with
increased costs of alternative sources of health insurance coverage." In addition, CBO found that
TRICARE beneficiaries use both inpatient and outpatient care at rates significantly higher than
people with other insurance, due to low out-of-pocket costs and other factors.

---

[22] Congressional Budget Office, *Long Term Implications of the 2013 Future Years Defense Program*, p. 21, http://www.cbo.gov/sites/default/files/cbofiles/attachments/07-11-12-FYDP_forPosting_0.pdf.

[23] Comptroller, Department of Defense. *National Defense Budget Estimates for FY2013*, March 2012. Table 5-5, Department of Defense Deflators–TOA. p. 60, http://comptroller.defense.gov/defbudget/fy2013/FY13_Green_Book.pdf.

Figure 4. CBO Depiction of Actual and Projected Costs for Military Health Care as a Share of DoD's Budget, 1990 to 2030

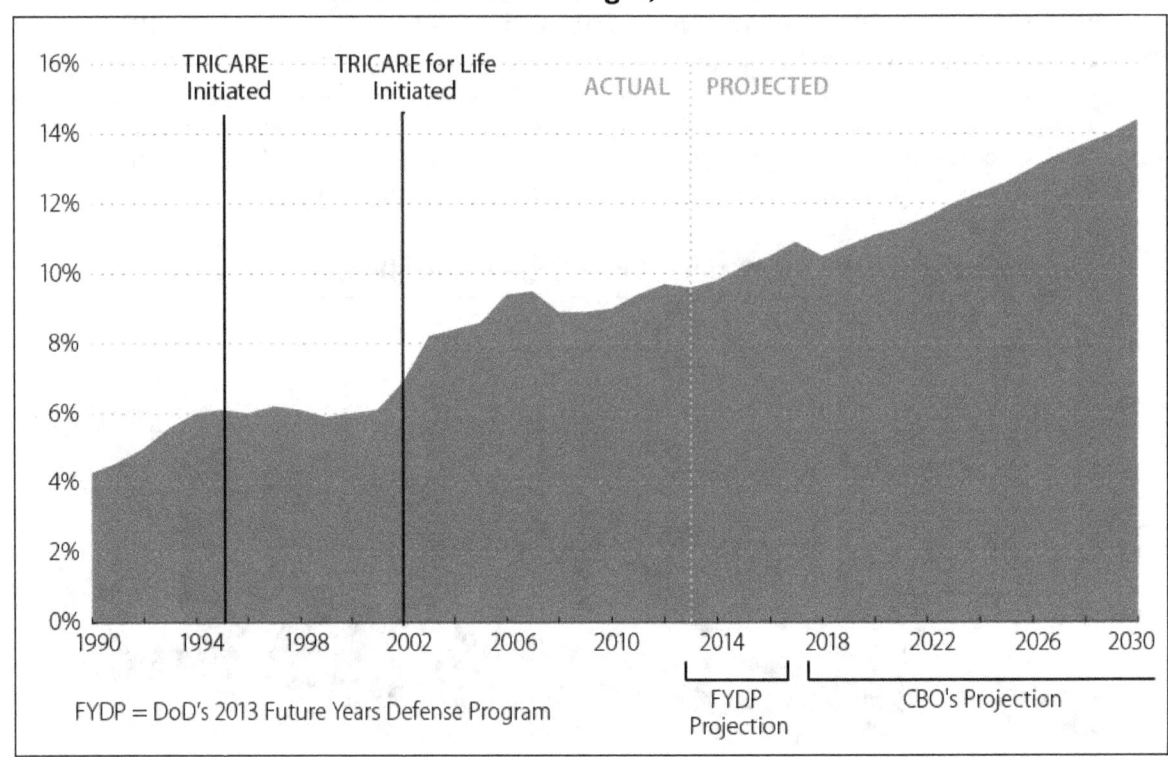

Source: Carla Tighe Murray, Approaches to Reduce Federal Spending on the Defense Health System, Congressional Budget Office, July 31, 2013, p. 2, http://www.cbo.gov/publication/44393.

DOD proposed new fees and cost-sharing increases for retiree TRICARE plans in their FY2013 budget submission. The new fee proposals were generally based on recommendations by the 2007 Task Force on the Future of Military Health Care. This congressionally created task force found that, "because costs borne by retirees under age 65 have been fixed in dollar terms since 1996, when TRICARE was being established, the portion of medical care costs assumed by these military retirees has declined by a factor of 2-3."[24] Overall, "military health care premiums paid by individual military retirees under age 65 utilizing DOD's most popular plan (TRICARE Prime) have fallen from 11% to 4%" of total health care costs.[25] These proposed cost-sharing increases and new fees were not adopted by the 112th Congress; however, as discussed above in "7. How Much Does Military Health Care Cost Beneficiaries?" above, some increases to pharmacy copayments were provided for in the National Defense Authorization Act for Fiscal Year 2013. The President's 2014 Budget also proposed new fee increases, however, none of these were adopted in the National Defense Authorization Act for Fiscal Year 2014.

---

[24] Department of Defense, subcommittee of the Defense Health Board, "Report of the Task Force on the Future of Military Health Care," December 2007, p. ES10, http://www.dcoe health.mil/Content/Navigation/Documents/103-06-2-Home-Task_Force_FINAL_REPORT_122007.pdf.

[25] Department of Defense, subcommittee of the Defense Health Board, "Report of the Task Force on the Future of Military Health Care," December 2007, p. 92, http://www.dcoe health mil/Content/Navigation/Documents/103-06-2-Home-Task_Force_FINAL_REPORT_122007.pdf.

12. How Does the Patient Protection and Affordable Care Act Affect TRICARE?

In general, the Patient Protection and Affordable Care Act (ACA)[26] does not directly affect TRICARE administration, health care benefits, eligibility, or cost to beneficiaries.[27]

Section 3110 of the ACA did open a special Medicare Part B enrollment window to enable certain individuals to gain coverage under the TRICARE for Life program.[28] The ACA also waived the Medicare Part B late enrollment penalty during the 12-month special enrollment period (SEP) for military retirees, their spouses (including widows/widowers), and dependent children who are otherwise eligible for TRICARE and are entitled to Medicare Part A based on disability or end-stage renal disease, but have declined Part B. The ACA required that the Secretary of Defense to identify and notify individuals of their eligibility for the SEP; the Secretary of Health and Human Services (HHS) and the Commissioner for Social Security support these efforts administratively. Section 3110 of the ACA was amended by the Medicare and Medicaid Extenders Act of 2010[29] to clarify that Section 3110 applies to Medicare Part B elections made on or after the date of enactment of the PPACA, which was on March 23, 2010.

13. How Are Private Health Care Providers Paid?

By law (P.L. 102-396) and Federal Regulation (32 CFR 199.14), health care providers treating TRICARE patients cannot bill for more than 115% of charges authorized by a DOD fee schedule. In some geographic areas, providers have been unwilling to accept TRICARE patients because of the limits on fees that can be charged. DOD has authority to grant exceptions. Statutes (10 U.S.C. 1079(h) and (j)) also require that payment levels for health care services provided under TRICARE be aligned with Medicare's fee schedule "to the extent practicable." Over 90% of TRICARE payment levels are now equivalent to those authorized by Medicare, about 10% are higher, and steps are being taken to adjust some to Medicare levels.

For institutional providers of outpatient services, TRICARE published a final regulation[30] that became effective on May 1, 2009, implementing the TRICARE outpatient prospective payment system (OPPS). Under 10 U.S.C. 1079(j)(2), DOD is required to use Medicare's reimbursement payment system for hospital outpatient services to the extent practicable. Under the OPPS, hospital outpatient services are paid on a rate-per-service basis that varies according to the Ambulatory Payment Classification (APC) group to which the services are assigned. Group services identified by Health Care Procedure Coding System (HCPCS) codes and descriptors within APC groups are the basis for setting payment rates under the hospital OPPS. To receive TRICARE reimbursement under the OPPS, providers must follow all Medicare specific coding requirements, except in those instances where the TRICARE Management Activity (TMA) develops specific APCs for those services that are unique to the TRICARE beneficiary

---

[26] P.L. 111-148.

[27] CRS Report R41198, *TRICARE and VA Health Care: Impact of the Patient Protection and Affordable Care Act (ACA)*, by Sidath Viranga Panangala and Don J. Jansen.

[28] §3110 of PPACA, P.L. 111-148.

[29] §201, P.L. 111-309.

[30] Department of Defense, "TRICARE: Outpatient Hospital Prospective Payment System (OPPS); Delay of Effective Date and Additional Opportunity for Public Comment," 74 *Federal Register* 6228, February 6, 2009.

population. For inpatient services, TMA regularly publishes reimbursement schedules through the Federal Register.

14. What Is the Relationship of DOD Health Care to Medicare?

TRICARE and Medicare Payments to Providers and the Sustainable Growth Rate

TRICARE is required to pay healthcare providers "to the extent practicable, in accordance with the same reimbursement rules as apply to payments for similar services"[31] under Medicare. This requirement was added by Section 731 of the National Defense Authorization Act for Fiscal Year 1996.[32]

The Sustainable Growth Rate (SGR) is the statutory method for determining the annual updates to the Medicare physician fee schedule, created in the Balanced Budget Act of 1997.[33] Under the SGR formula, "if [Medicare] expenditures over a period are less than the cumulative spending target for the period, the annual update [to the provider fee schedule] is increased. However, if spending exceeds the cumulative spending target over a certain period, future updates are reduced to bring spending back in line with the target."[34] In other words, if Medicare costs are greater than expected, the provider fees are reduced to bring overall Medicare expenditures down towards expected levels.[35]

Each year since 2002, the SGR system has produced a formula result, "conversion factor" that would reduce reimbursement rates. With the exception of 2002, when a 4.8% decrease was applied, Congress has overridden the SGR formula-driven reductions to provider fee rates through a series of temporary postponements known as "doc fixes."

Most recently, the Pathway for SGR Reform Act of 2013 (§1101 of H.J.Res. 59) overrode the SGR formula-driven reimbursement rates until March 31, 2014. The most recent calculation of the cut in reimbursement rates that would have occurred absent an override was 23.7%.[36]

Although the law requires TRICARE reimbursement rates to be equal to Medicare rates "to the extent practicable," it does permit TRICARE to make exceptions to ensure an adequate network of providers or to eliminate a situation of severely impaired access to care.

---

[31] 10 U.S.C. 1079.

[32] P.L. 104-106.

[33] P.L. 105-33.

[34] See §1848 of the Social Security Act codified at 42 U.S.C. 1395w–4.

[35] For more information on the SGR please see: CRS Report R40907, *Medicare Physician Payment Updates and the Sustainable Growth Rate (SGR) System*, by Jim Hahn and Janemarie Mulvey.

[36] Congressional Budget Office, *Medicare's*, December 6, 2013, p. Note a., http://www.cbo.gov/sites/default/files/cbofiles/attachments/2013%20SGR%20Options%20-%20Final%20Rule.pdf.

Medicare and TRICARE for Life

Active duty military personnel have been fully covered by Social Security and have paid Social Security taxes since January 1, 1957. In 1965, Congress created Medicare under Title 18 of the Social Security Act to provide health insurance to people age 65 and older, regardless of income or medical history. Social Security coverage includes eligibility for health care coverage under Medicare at age 65.

In establishing CHAMPUS in 1966, it was the legislative intent of Congress that retired members of the uniformed services and their eligible dependents be provided with medical care after they retire from the military, usually between their late-30s and mid-40s. However, Congress did not intend that CHAMPUS should replace Medicare as a supplemental benefit to military health care. For this reason, retirees became ineligible to receive CHAMPUS benefits when, at age 65, they become eligible for Medicare.

Many argued that the structure was inherently unfair because retirees lost TRICARE/CHAMPUS benefits at the stage in life when they were increasingly likely to need them. It was argued that military personnel had been promised free medical care for life, not just until age 65. After considerable debate over various options for ensuring medical care to retired beneficiaries, Congress in the Floyd D. Spence National Defense Authorization Act for Fiscal Year 2001[37] provided that, beginning October 1, 2001, TRICARE would pay out-of-pocket costs for services provided under Medicare for beneficiaries over age 64 if they are enrolled in Medicare Part B. This benefit is known as TRICARE for Life (TFL). Disabled persons under age 65 who are entitled to Medicare may continue to receive CHAMPUS benefits as a secondary payer to Medicare Parts A and B (with some restrictions).

The requirement for enrollment in Medicare Part B, which has typical premiums of $104.90 per month in 2013,[38] is a source of concern to some beneficiaries, especially those who did not enroll in Part B when they became 65 and thus must pay significant penalties. Some argue that this requirement is unfair since Part B enrollment was not originally a prerequisite for access to any DOD medical care. On the other hand, waiving the penalty for military retirees could be considered unfair to other Medicare-users who did not enroll in Part B upon turning 65. The Medicare Prescription Drug, Improvement, and Modernization Act[39] (P.L. 108-173), passed in December 2003, waived penalties for military retirees in certain circumstances during an open season in 2004.[40] More recently, the ACA created another special enrollment period. (See question #12).

15. What Medical Benefits are Available to Reservists?

Reservists and National Guardsmen (members of the "Reserve Component") who are serving on active duty have the same medical benefits as regular military personnel. Reserve personnel while on active duty for training and during weekly or monthly drills also are covered for illnesses

---

[37] P.L. 106-398.

[38] CRS Report R40082, *Medicare: Part B Premiums*, by Patricia A. Davis.

[39] P.L. 108-173.

[40] See out-of-print CRS Report RS21731, *Medicare: Part B Premium Penalty*, by Jennifer O'Sullivan, available upon request.

incurred while on training or traveling to or from their duty station. In recent years, especially as members of the Reserve Component have had a larger role in combat operations overseas, Congress has broadened the medical benefits available for Reservists. Those who have been notified that they are to be activated are now covered by TRICARE up to 180 days before reporting. Reservists who have served more than 30 days after having been called up for active duty in a contingency operation are eligible for 180 days of TRICARE coverage after the end of their service under the Transitional Assistance Management Program (TAMP). In addition, the TRICARE Reserve Select (TRS) program is an optional program available to Reserve Component members while not activated. To be eligible for TRS, the member must not be on active duty orders, not be covered under the Transitional Assistance Management Program, and not be eligible for or enrolled in the Federal Employees Health Benefits Program. TRS coverage requires payment of monthly premiums (in 2013, $51.62 for individual coverage, $195.81 for member and family coverage).

16. Have Military Personnel Been Promised Free Medical Care for Life?

Some military personnel and former military personnel maintain that they and their dependents were promised "free medical care for life" at the time of their enlistment. Such promises may have been made by military recruiters and in recruiting brochures; however, if they were made, they were not based upon laws or official regulations, which provide only for access to military medical facilities for non-active-duty personnel if space is available as described above. Space was not always available and TRICARE options could involve significant costs to beneficiaries. Rear Admiral Harold M. Koenig, the Deputy Assistant Secretary of Defense for Health Affairs, testified in May 1993: "We have a medical care program for life for our beneficiaries, and it is pretty well defined in the law. That easily gets interpreted to, or reinterpreted into, free medical care for the rest of your life. That is a pretty easy transition for people to make in their thinking, and it is pervasive. We [DOD] spend an incredible amount of effort trying to re-educate people [that] that is not their benefit."[41]

Dr. Stephen C. Joseph, Assistant Secretary of Defense for Health Affairs in April 1998, however, argued that because retirees believe they have had a promise of free care, the government did have an obligation. Joseph did not specify the precise extent of the obligation. The FY1998 Defense Authorization Act (P.L. 105-85) included (in Section 752) a finding that "many retired military personnel believe that they were promised lifetime health care in exchange for 20 or more years of service," and expressed the sense of Congress that "the United States has incurred a moral obligation to provide health care to members and [retired] members of the Armed Services." Further, it is necessary "to provide quality, affordable care to such retirees."

---

[41] U.S. Congress, House of Representatives, Committee on Armed Services, Military Forces and Personnel Subcommittee, 103rd Congress, 1st session, *National Defense Authorization Act for Fiscal Year 1994—H.R. 2401 and Oversight of Previously Authorized Programs*, Hearings, H.A.S.C. No. 103-13, April 27, 28, May 10, 11, and 13, 1993, p. 505.

17. What is the Congressionally Directed Medical Research Program?

Many different entities within the Department of Defense request appropriations for and are funded to conduct a wide range of medical research. Over the last 17 years, Congress has supplemented the DOD appropriations to include additional unrequested funding for specific medical research funding. In 1992, Congress appropriated $25 million for breast cancer research to be managed by DOD's U.S. Army Medical Research and Materiel Command (USAMRMC). The following year, Congress appropriated $210 million to the DOD for extramural, peer-reviewed breast cancer research.

Following this, DOD established the Congressionally Directed Medical Research Programs (CDMRP) within USAMRMC. The Program now manages congressionally directed appropriations totaling $6 billion through FY2010 for research on breast, prostate, and ovarian cancers; neurofibromatosis; military health; chronic myelogenous leukemia; tuberous sclerosis complex; autism; psychological health and traumatic brain injury; amyotrophic lateral sclerosis; Gulf War Illness; deployment-related health research; and other health concerns.[42] This additional, unrequested funding now appears in the Defense Health Program RDT&E appropriation. Conference report language usually includes a table instructing DOD on how to allocate the additional funding to specific diseases and research areas. This guidance is not considered to be an earmark because the funding is used for peer-reviewed, competitively awarded research grants.

Table 2 depicts appropriations for selected CDMRP programs.

Table 2. Appropriation Levels by Fiscal Year (FY) for Selected CDMR Programs, FY2007-FY2013

(in millions of current dollars)

	FY2007[a]	FY2008[b]	FY2009[c]	FY2010[d]	FY2011[e]	FY2012[f]	FY2013
Amyotrophic Lateral Sclerosis	5	0	5	7.5	8	6.4	7.5
Autism	7.5	6.4	8	8	6.4	5.1	6.0
Bone Marrow Failure	0	0	5	3.75	4	3.2	3.2
Breast Cancer/Breast Cancer Research	127.5	138	150	150	150	120	120
Gulf War Illness	0	10	8	8	8	10	20
Lung Cancer	0	0	20	15	12.8	10.2	120
Multiple Sclerosis	0	0	5	4.5	4.8	3.8	5
Neurofibromatosis	10	8	10	13.75	16	12.8	15
Ovarian Cancer	10	10	20	18.75	20	16	20

---

[42] Department of Defense, *Congressionally Directed Medical Research Program: FY 2008 Annual Report*, September 30, 2008, pp. 1-2, http://cdmrp.army mil/annreports/2008annrep/default htm.

	FY2007[a]	FY2008[b]	FY2009[c]	FY2010[d]	FY2011[e]	FY2012[f]	FY2013
Peer-Reviewed Cancer	0	0	16	15	16	12.8	15
Peer-Reviewed Medical	0	50	50	50	50	50	50
Peer-Reviewed Orthopedic	0	0	51	22.5	24	30	30
Prostate Cancer	80	80	80	80	80	80	80
Psychological Health/Traumatic Brain Injury	150	0	165	120	100	135.5	135
Spinal Cord Injury	0	0	35	11.25	12	9.6	30
Tuberous Sclerosis	0	4	6	6	6.4	5.1	6

Source: Congressionally Directed Medical Research Program, Annual Reports FY2007–FY2012, Recommendations accompanying the Defense Appropriations Acts.

Notes:

a. Funds appropriated by P.L. 110-5 (see H.Rept. 109-676 to H.R. 5631, September 25, 2006, pages 248-250), http://www.gpo.gov/fdsys/pkg/CRPT-109hrpt676/pdf/CRPT-109hrpt676.pdf.

b. Funds appropriated by P.L. 110-116. See *Congressional Record*, November 6, 2007, p. H13119.

c. Funds appropriated by Division C of P.L. 110-329. See *Congressional Record*, September 24, 2008, pp. H9725–H9726.

d. Funds appropriated by P.L. 111-117. See *Congressional Record*, December 16, 2009, p. H15319–H15320, http://www.gpo.gov/fdsys/pkg/CREC-2009-12-16/pdf/CREC-2009-12-16-pt1-PgH15007-2.pdf#page=314.

e. Funds appropriated by P.L. 112-10. See House Rules Committee' tables accompanying H.R. 1473, pp. 53-54, http://rules.house.gov/Media/file/FY11-Defense-Department-Base-tables.pdf.

f. Funds appropriated by P.L. 112-74 (H.R. 2055). See House Rules Committee's tables accompanying H.R. 2055, 92A, p. 282, http://rules.house.gov/Media/file/PDF_112_1/legislativetext/H.R.2055crSOM/psConference%20Div%20A%20-%20SOM%20OCR.pdf.

g. Funds appropriated by P.L. 113-6 (H.R. 933). Figures not adjusted for sequestration reductions of 7.95%. See Senate Explanation Statement, p. S1515 at http://www.gpo.gov/fdsys/pkg/CREC-2013-03-11/pdf/CREC-2013-03-11-pt1-PgS1287.pdf#page=1.

The CDMRP website (http://cdmrp.army.mil/) also provides specific descriptions and funding histories of the different research programs.

18. Other Frequently Asked Questions

Does TRICARE Cover Abortion?

10 U.S.C. 1093 provides that "Funds available to the Department of Defense may not be used to perform abortions except where the life of the mother would be endangered if the fetus were carried to term or in a case in which the pregnancy is the result of an act of rape or incest."[43]

---

[43] The clause "or in a case in which the pregnancy is the result of an act of rape or incest" was added by Section 704 of the National Defense Authorization Act for Fiscal Year 2013.

Does DOD Use Animals in Medical Research or Training?

Yes. DOD policy is that live animals will not be used for training and education except where, after exhaustive analysis, no alternatives are available. Currently approved uses include pre-deployment training for medical personnel and include infant intubation (ferrets); microsurgery (rodents); and combat trauma training (goats and swine).

Author Contact Information

Don J. Jansen
Analyst in Defense Health Care Policy
djansen@crs.loc.gov, 7-4769